Don't Count
Me Out Yet

Don't Count Me Out Yet

Eleanor M. Newby

To order additional copies of this book, contact:
Xlibris Corporation
1-888-795-4274
www.Xlibris.com
Orders@Xlibris.com
89982

CONTENTS

Dedicated to my Lord and Savior, Jesus Christ, who gave me the gift of writing and for helping me through all the battles, especially the one I have had since 2003. Without Him giving me the strength to be here and for opening doors, this book would not be possible.

ACKNOWLEDGEMENTS

This book has taken me almost three years to write. I have always loved to write and I have always kept a journal. The journal really came in handy when I had to remember dates for the book. There are so many people I need to thank and I hope I don't leave anyone out. If I do, please forgive me and know it was not intentional. I dedicated this book to my Lord and Savior, Jesus Christ, but I feel I need to thank Him again for being the most important person in my life.

A special thanks to my husband, Roy, whom I was married to for **41** years. Thank you to my precious boys, Randy and Rusty and their wives, Hilary and Bridget. Thank you for giving me the most precious gift you could have ever given me, my grandchildren, Sydney, Laney, and Ryan Zane. They are the joy of my life. Thank you to my sisters, Edna, Hazel, and Joyce. Thank you to all my nieces, nephews, cousins, brother-in-laws. Thank you, Angie and Dean, Skyler, Cameron, Brennen, and Zoe.

A special thanks to my oncologist, Dr. Harry McCoy, my radiation doctor, Dr. Ojomo, and to all my nurses and caregivers. I would like to name them all, but you know who you are. Thank you to all my physical therapists and doctors and especially Dr. Russell Melton, who sent me to a surgeon when I first saw him and suspected that I did have cancer.

Thank you to all my friends at Celco that I worked with over the years, especially Tony and Doris who were there for me when I first went back to work after my diagnosis. Thanks for all the concern shown to me by my other friends at work and for all my bosses who always cared how I was feeling.

Thank you to all my friends who took me to my chemo and radiation treatments. A special thanks to my sister, Joyce who has been a rock for me over the years, even though she is the youngest. And Madeline, my special friend, I could never thank you enough for always being there for me. I hope I have been half as good a friend to you as you have been to me.

Thank you for all the people and teachers over the years who encouraged me and saw my potential. Thank you especially to those who encouraged me to go to college even later in life and work towards a goal.

Thank you to all my church family at Cornerstone, especially to my pastors, John and Millie Jenkins. Thank you to my friend and music leader, Terri, who has always encouraged me to use my talents to sing and play music. Thank you to Pastor David Roberts, although he doesn't know it, the inspiration for this book came to me when he was teaching us the class about "The Dreamgiver."

Thank you for all the people who have touched my life in any way and to my friends who have gone through this same battle and many of them lost. I know I will see all of you again someday.

Thanks again to my loving husband, Roy, who although he is no longer with me, I still feel his presence and know he is still taking care of me. No one could ever know how much I miss him, but I know I must go on for my family and friends.

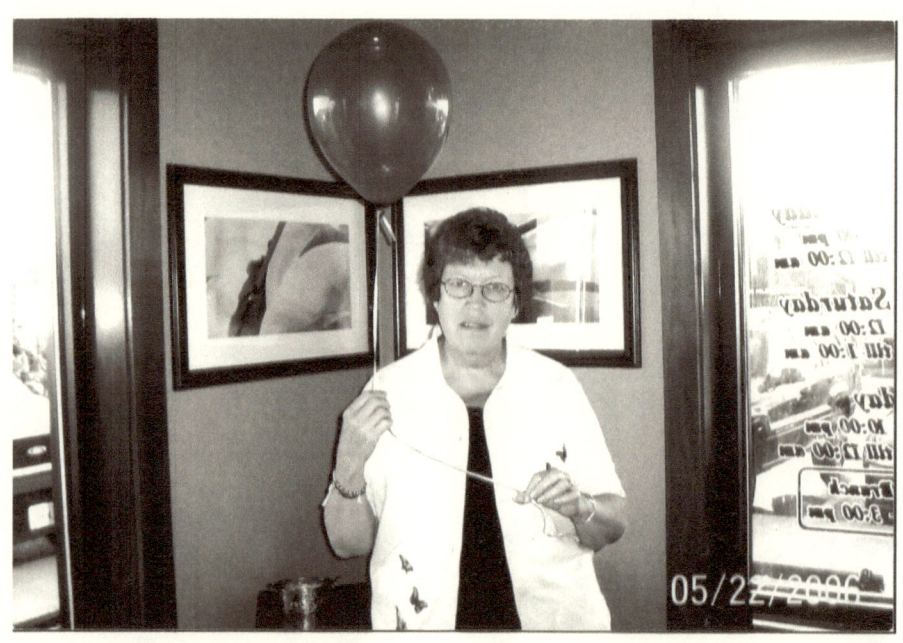

Myself

Chapter I

"In the Beginning"

My life began in a little town called Bluff City, Virginia. I was to be the next to last child Mom had. I was one of six children. I had an older brother, two older sisters, a younger brother and a younger sister. My youngest brother died at about sixteen months of age from meningitis. We never knew him or even saw a picture of him. Money was tight back then and evidently there were no pictures. Mom told me he had red hair. It ran in our family and I would later have a red-headed son that Mom told me looked a lot like my brother we lost. Mom had me and my younger sister late in life. She was forty when she had me and forty-five when she had my youngest sister, Joyce. Back then, a lot of children were born at home which was the case for all of us except Joyce. She was the only one born in a hospital. I can't imagine giving birth at home without all the modern equipment and drugs we have today, especially when there are complications.

We didn't have a lot growing up, but we always felt like we had the things we needed. Dad was out of work a lot and we wore hand-me-downs and got a lot of help from friends and our older siblings when they left home and got married. I don't ever remember being hungry or doing without and we never expected things other children had. Once in a while, when Dad was working, we got a doll or some toy we wanted. We never felt deprived because our family was close and we loved each other.

I was able to finish high school with good grades and I also worked the last two years of high school at a little drugstore in Narrows, Virginia called "Little Doc's Cut Rate." I really thought I was something being a working girl and having spending money. I also got a discount on anything I bought in the store. I didn't make a lot of money back then, but I felt privileged to be able to buy a new blouse or a pair of shoes. I can remember my first pair of shoes I bought. They were a little too big because they didn't have my size, but I stuffed tissues in the toe and wore them anyway. They were plain black loafers, (not the penny kind), and every day after I had worn them, I wiped them off and put them back in the box.

Eventually I got married and had a family and then my youngest sister got married. I worked a lot of different jobs, but in 1967, I got on at a local factory called the Celanese and I worked there 37 years until my retirement.

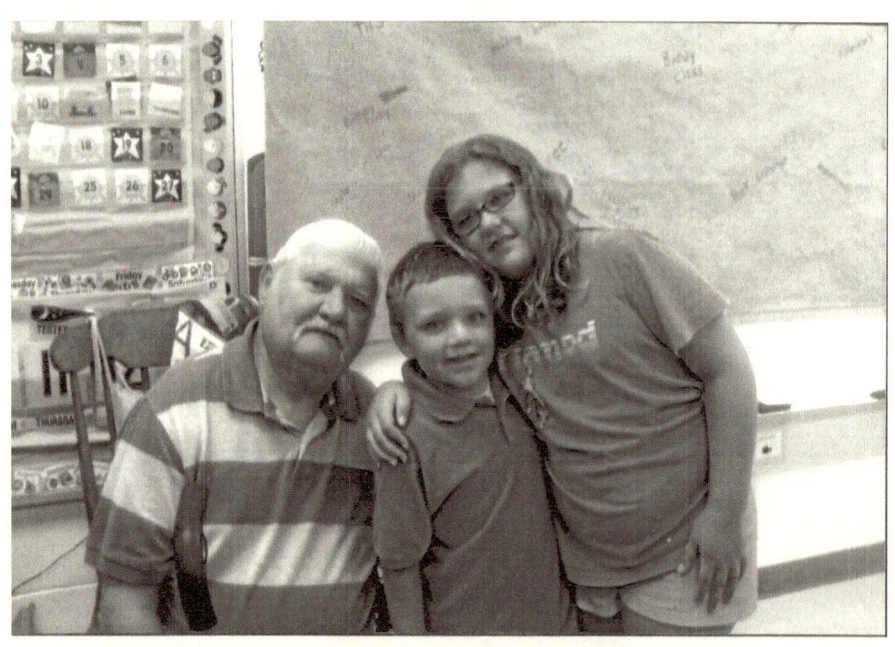

PAW-PAW (My Roy), Ryan and Laney.
Ryan's Kindergarten Graduation 2008.

Chapter II

"A Bad Year"

You know how you hear people say, "That was a good year." I've had many good years in my life-graduation, getting my job, getting married, the birth of my children and the birth of each of my grandchildren. I've also had some years not so good. 1996 was one of them. My husband of 28 years had a heart attack and then had to have open-heart surgery. I turned 50 that year and my youngest son went into the military. He was only 21 and I thought my heart would break. Most of the time, the oldest child leaves first, but as it turned out, Rusty went from graduation from high school to working and going to college part-time to getting married. Randy, on the other hand, stayed with us longer before he moved out, got married and started his family. I remember one Christmas, while Rusty was in the Army and he was in Seoul, South Korea. I didn't want to make a big deal about it because Randy was still home, so I didn't say anything, but he did. He said, "It just doesn't seem the same without Rusty." He was feeling the same thing. The boys fought a lot when they were small, as most siblings do, but they are very close. It was hard after the boys left home and I had the empty nest syndrome for a while, but I had to believe we had raised them both the right way and they were adults and could make it through life just fine. I survived with the boys gone and life was pretty good until things really started happening in 2000.

January 25, 2000, I got a phone call that my nephew, Travis had been in a car wreck with two other boys. I would later find out that he and the boy driving were killed instantly and the other boy was flown to Roanoke where he later died, too. His name was David and he left behind a wife who was pregnant with their first child. She would have him just a few days later and name him after his Dad. This was a son he would never get to see. Travis and Lee were not married, but there were three families torn apart. The boys were out joy riding and ran under a dump truck. We still believe they never saw the truck, because the road they were killed on was just a straight stretch of highway. Travis was my youngest sister's only son and he had an older sister, Angie, who was married and had a son, Skyler who always looked up to Travis and called him Tat-Tay. This was one of the hardest times in my life, losing him. I had lost my Dad in 1983. It was hard, but he was almost 80 and had heart trouble and cancer, so we were expecting it. He died at the VA Hospital in Salem, Virginia.

After Daddy died, Mom came to live with me because she had never really been alone. My other sisters helped me, but she made her home with me. She was in fairly good health when she came to live with m and I would have her for 15 years.

Then in 2002, she started experiencing some problems. She would see things that weren't there and she would talk out of her head sometimes for a day or two and then sleep for a day or two. Our local doctor would come to the house and check her and up until now, she seemed to be doing all right. He had her on heart medicine and sometimes he gave her medicine for her nerves.

I came in from work one day and my husband told me she had fallen out of bed, and he had put her back, but I better check on her. I did and she seemed fine except she seemed to be having some pain. I took her to the emergency room, and they checked her and x-rayed her and sent her home. It was a relief she had no broken bones, and I thought she would bounce back as she had done so many times in the past.

After a couple of days, she seemed to get worse and she was unable to get out of bed. My sisters would come and help feed her and bathe her, but she was almost helpless. Her appetite decreased and I would have her sit up in bed as I fed her and she would sometimes fall over. I knew I would have to call the doctor to come check her, but I couldn't even think of the possibility of putting her in a nursing home or even worse, losing her.

When the doctor came to check her, he sat at the kitchen table with me to discuss his diagnosis. I told him I needed help with her and he told me he was going to get me some help. It was getting so hard for my sisters and me and we were afraid she needed more help than we could give her. He looked at me with a serious look on his face and told me that Mom was terminal. I certainly wasn't expecting to hear that word. He said she had dementia, which is a form of Alzheimer's. He set me up with the hospice people and they began to come each day to bathe her and feed her and make up her bed. We got her a hospital bed, and had oxygen available in case she ever needed it. Even though I was so thankful for the help, and her spirits seemed to lift with the extra attention, I still couldn't accept the possibility of losing her.

As much as I hated to admit it, I saw her health decline and on November 30th, with all of us around her, she died with a beautiful smile on her face. I am so thankful she died so peacefully with her family by her bedside.

Little did I know that just a few months later, we would go through heartache again with the loss of my mother-in-law. She went into the hospital for surgery for an aortic aneurysm, which we knew, was risky. She made it though the surgery and we went to see her and told her she could come and stay with us after she got out of the hospital. Just a few days later she contacted necro facilitis, which is known as the flesh eating disease, and we lost her too. My boys lost both their grandmothers within a matter of a few months. The only bright spot out of all of this was the birth of our first grandson, Ryan, born only one day after we lost Maw-Maw.

Losing my Mom was one of the hardest things I had to endure in my life. I had been so used to having her around. I have to admit it got hard at times, but I wouldn't take back one minute of time I sacrificed to take care of her. I know she is in heaven now with Dad and other loved ones, but I still miss her a lot. I still see her sometimes with that beautiful smile she always had. That was one of the first things you noticed about her. She was always concerned more about her family than she was about herself. She taught me about the Lord and to be honest and to help other people and that is one thing I have always carried in my life.

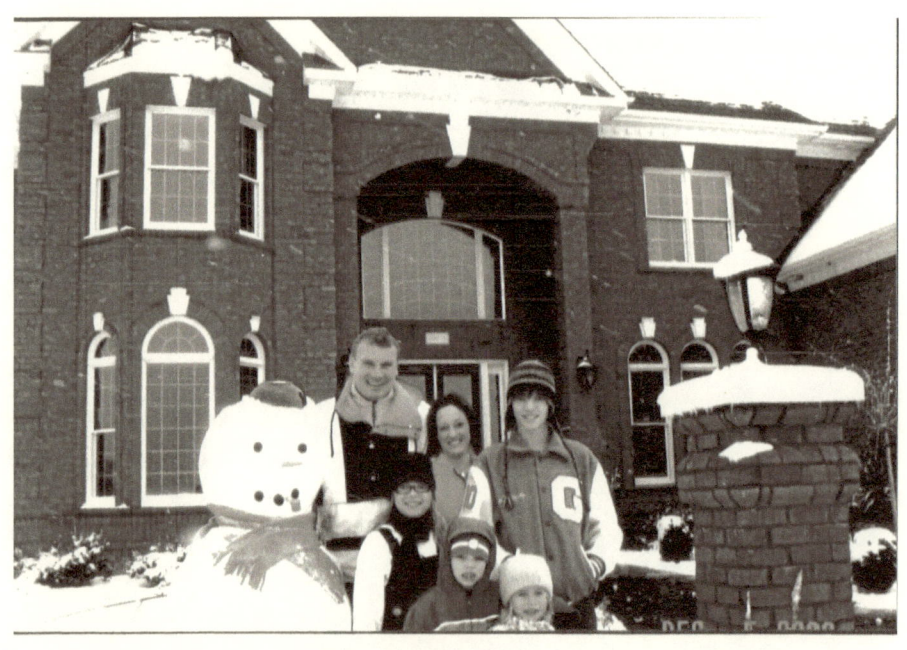

Dean, Angie, Skyler, Cameron, Brennen and Zoe in front of their house, Winter 2009.

CHAPTER III

"Facing The Battle"

Sometimes when you look back on things and wonder why they happened, I know now God was getting me prepared for a great battle that was lying ahead for me. I know now it would have been impossible for me to continue to care for Mom and deal with what I was getting ready to go through. I also have a peace in my heart that she is not suffering any more. She lived for 95 years and that is a great testimony in itself.

In July, 2003, my life seemed to be going good. I had been married to the same man for 35 years and we had two grown sons and three beautiful grandchildren. My oldest son, Randy and his wife, Hilary had a little boy, Ryan and my youngest son, Rusty and his wife, Bridget, had two girls, Sydney and Laney. They all had good jobs and this was certainly a blessing. I had worked at the same production plant for 37 years and was considering early retirement. Because of a history of breast cancer in my family, (a sister and an aunt), I tried to have a mammogram every year when I had my yearly physical. I had one in December of 2002 and when I got the results, everything seemed fine. Here it was about seven months later and I was getting ready to go to work on the 11-7 shift. As I got out of the shower, I was standing looking in the mirror and I noticed my nipple on my left breast looked like it was inverted. It didn't alarm me too much, but I decided to be on the safe side I would call my family doctor the next day and make an appointment and have it checked out.

The next day I came in from work and stayed up until the doctor's office opened and called and made an appointment. Then I went to bed and tried to get some sleep and not worry too much. I had a strong faith and I prayed everything would be all right. When I got up, I got ready and went to keep my appointment. They asked the usual questions, and then I went in to see the doctor. I told him my concerns, and after examining me, he asked me if I had been sick recently. I told him I had had a virus that was going around, but I was feeling better. He told me I might have an infection in my breast and he was going to put me on antibiotics. He also told me to come back in two weeks. I left, feeling better and hoped the medicine would take care of everything.

I took the antibiotics, but my breast seemed to be getting worse. It got really red and inflamed and sore. I really started getting concerned then. In the past I had lumps removed several times, and they all turned out to be benign, but I had never experienced anything like I was experiencing now. I kept my appointment and went back in two weeks. After checking me again, I could tell the doctor was concerned. He told me with my history, he thought it would be a good idea for me to see a surgeon. He suggested one to me in Blacksburg and had his nurse make me an appointment. Before I went to see him, my breast seemed to be getting worse. It was so hard and it felt hot to the touch and seemed to be getting hard and swollen.

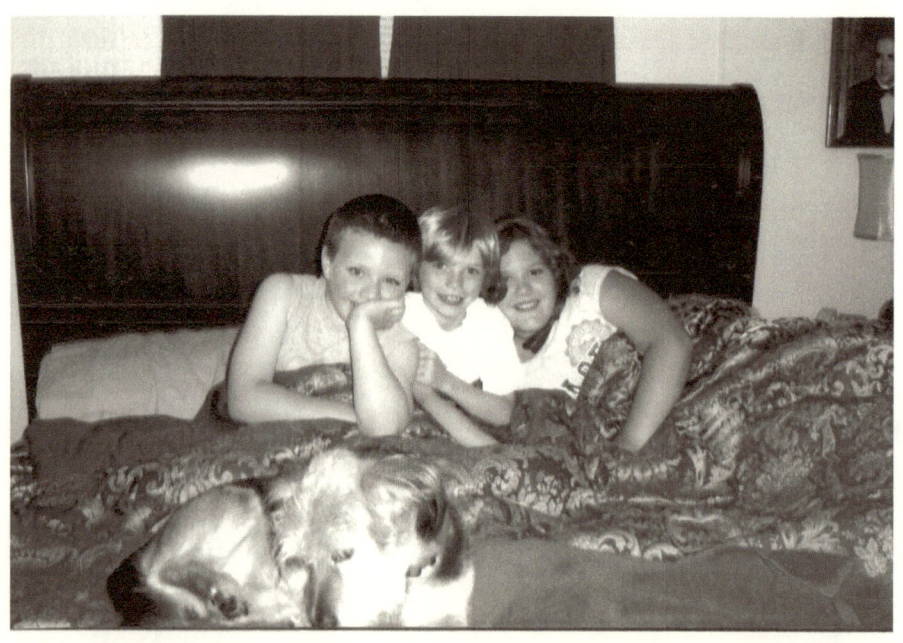

Ryan, Brennen, Laney and "Biscuit" at Joyce's house in her big bed.

Chapter IV

"The Diagnosis"

The day of my appointment, my husband went with me. The nurse came in and took my history and told me to undress and get on a gown and wait for the doctor to see me. She also asked me why I was there. After she left, I got undressed and put on the gown. It seemed like an eternity before the doctor came in to see me. As he entered he shook my hand, asked me how I was doing and seemed very nice. I explained to him the problems I had been having and he told me to lie down on the table and he would check me.

He checked my right breast first, and then my left. I could tell by the look on his face, he was concerned. He told me he couldn't be sure without a biopsy, but he was pretty sure I had invasive ductal carcinoma. I didn't understand all of the medical terms he used, but I knew carcinoma was cancer. My heart fell. He then told me they would go ahead and do the biopsy in the office. He left the room and had his nurse to prepare me for the biopsy.

She put some medicine on my chest. Soon he returned to the room and told me he was going to insert a needle into my breast to numb it. He proceeded to do this and it was painful, but I was hoping it would numb my breast enough that the biopsy wouldn't be too bad. As he was inserting the needle, I could tell he was having a hard time inserting it all the way into my breast. I found out later that was because the tumor was so large and my breast had become really hard. He waited a few minutes and then inserted another instrument into the side of my breast for the biopsy. This really hurt. It was especially painful because the numbing medicine had not gotten all the way into that area. I tried to take deep breaths and he kept asking if I was all right. I told him yes. I wanted to get this over with and find out the results as soon as possible. He took about six or seven tissue samples and after what seemed like an eternity, he was finished. He then put in a few stitches and left the room. He told me if I would hang around for a while that the pathologist was coming by and they would be able to give me the results of my biopsy. I told him I would wait because I wanted to find out the results, good or bad, that day. He left the room. The nurse cleaned my chest off and put a bandage on it and then she left and told me she would check on me in a few minutes.

After they both left, so many things were going through my mind. I really felt deep down that the news wouldn't be good and I knew I had to face what lie ahead and do whatever it took to prolong my life as long as I could. I tried to imagine life with my breast gone, but I had talked to other friends who had gone through this, and they seemed to be doing fine.

He finally returned to the room. I had gotten off the table and was sitting in a chair and he rolled his little stool over to me and looked me straight in the eye. He told me it was bad and I needed to have surgery right away. I knew he didn't mean a lumpectomy but he meant a mastectomy. A feeling came over me I can't explain, but those of you who have been there know what I was feeling. He wanted me to have surgery that week, but I told him my husband was diagnosed with an abdominal aortic aneurysm and he was scheduled for major surgery in Charlottesville that week. He said he would schedule mine for the next week.

Some of my friends and family would later question why I waited for a week, but I knew I couldn't let my husband go through his surgery without me, because he would be worried about me and I would be worried about him. I have never regretted my decision.

When I returned to the waiting room, I told him what the doctor had told me and I could tell by the look on his face, it was very disturbing to him. I knew he would have a lot of questions and I waited until we were on our way home to answer them. I told him everything and that I was going to wait and have my surgery after he got through his. He said I didn't have to wait, but I knew secretly he was glad I was going to be with him during his surgery. It seemed like a double whammy. We had already been through the pain of losing our mothers within months of each other and now we were facing another battle that we would have to go through together.

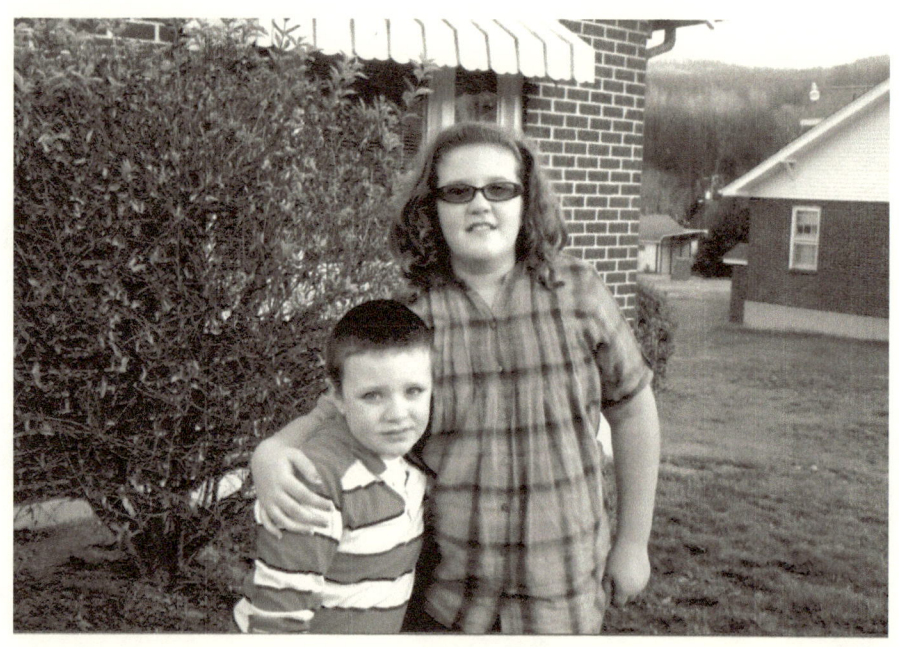

Laney and Ryan, Thanksgiving 2010.

Chapter V

"Facing Another Battle"

Soon came time for our trip to Charlottesville. I woke up that day not feeling too well. I drank a cup of coffee and we packed some bags because we knew we would be at least staying overnight. We picked up my sister, Joyce, and proceeded to go to the hospital. It is about a three and a half or four-hour drive if you don't run into traffic or a wreck on the way. My husband always likes to leave early for any doctor appointments we have out of town. I was so glad to have my sister with me. It makes things so much easier and she and my husband have a good relationship.

Finally we reached the hospital and got him checked in. I saw my husband whisper something to my sister and she came and told me I had blood on the back of my pants. My first thought was my cancer was worse than I thought and I had waited too long. I knew they were probably thinking the same thing. She went out to the car to get me a change of clothes and I went in the bathroom and changed. After a while, I knew the bleeding had come from a problem I had had for years which was hemorrhoids. Up in the day, I started feeling better and stopped worrying about myself and concentrated on my husband's upcoming surgery.

He came through the surgery all right and we returned home the next day. He was very sore and I took care of him the best I could. He had a stent inserted into his abdomen. Actually, we had to make several trips to Charlottesville over the next year. He wound up with five stents, one on either side of his groin and the others in his abdomen. They were all done at different times and the doctors told us his was one of the most complicated surgeries they had ever done.

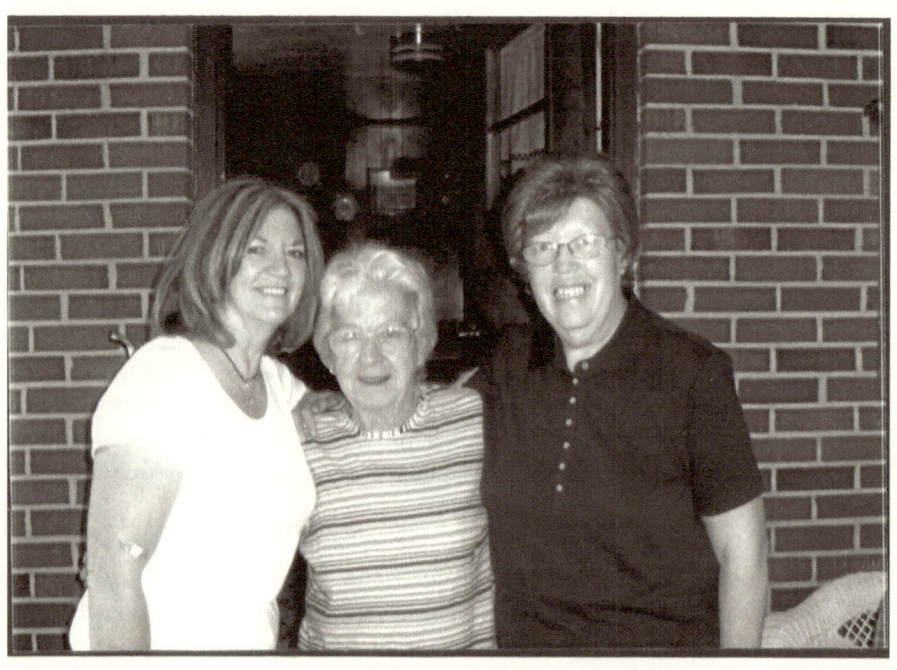

Me, Hazel and Joyce.
Hazel's house May 2010.

Chapter VI

"Going Into Surgery"

I waited on him that week and soon it was time for me to go to the hospital for my surgery. I asked Roy not to go with me. I told him he could come over later. I didn't want him to have to sit all day. He was still really sore and recuperating from his surgery. My sister, Joyce came and got me and took me to the hospital. I had already pre-registered the day before so after we got there; they took me into a room and started preparing me for my surgery. My pastor came over and other friends from chuch and they all prayed with me before they took me downstairs.

They had already started some i.v. and the anesthesiologist came and told me how he was going to give me medicine to put me to sleep. My surgeon had already been in to talk to me and explain all that was involved in the surgery. He told me if any lymph nodes looked suspicious, he would remove them too. As the medicine started to work, I soon was asleep. The next thing I knew, they were trying to wake me up and the surgery was over. I was in some pain, but they were really good to ask me if I needed anything. I stayed in the recovery room for about an hour. Then they took me up to my room. My husband had come over with our youngest son and my sister was still there. I had many visitors that night. Of course, you can't remember everyone because you are still groggy from the surgery and the pain medicine they are still giving you. The doctor came in and told me my tumor was so large that it had completely taken over my breast. He had to cut deep into my chest to remove it all and it had weighed seven pounds. He had also removed 16 lymph nodes and he would tell me later if they were malignant. He told me I had to stay at least overnight and he would check on me the next morning. I couldn't get up the first night and my blood pressure was very low. They checked me often and it remained low through the night. They told me part of the reason was because of the morphine I was on and the other reason was because I couldn't get up yet. They told me it would probably start coming back up the next day after they got me up. My sister stayed the night. She was afraid to leave me. She curled up in a little ball and slept in a chair.

The doctor came in the next day and asked me if I wanted to go home and I said yes. I knew it would be hard for me when I returned home because my husband was still recovering from surgery and he certainly couldn't wait on me.

My cousin and her husband, who were in visiting from Culpeper, VA, came to pick me up and take me home. I was so glad to get home. They stayed for a while, and then they returned to my sister's house where they were staying until they returned to Culpeper.

Chapter VIII

"Preparing for Treatments"

Before I started my chemo treatments, I had to go into the hospital as an out-patient and have a portacath inserted in my chest. This would be done by my surgeon. This would make it easier for the nurses to access for my chemo and also to draw blood. Chemo is very hard on your veins and I would see in the months ahead, this portacath would be a lifesaver for me in so many ways. I had this procedure done, and I was a little sore for a few days, but other than a little lump in my skin, I soon forgot it was there.

When I went to visit my oncologist, he would explain to me exactly what we were dealing with and what options there were. His name was Dr. McCoy and I loved him the first time we met. He had such a gentle nature and I knew when he looked into my eyes that he would be someone I could trust. I didn't have much choice. After all, I was putting my life into his hands. I believe first we have to trust God for our healing, but I also believe he puts us with good doctors and nurses to help us through our battles.

He sat down and took my hand. He had my chart in his hand and had gone over everything that my surgeon had sent to him. He looked me right in the eye and told me I had inflammatory breast cancer. This was a medical term I had never heard before. He told me it was a very invasive type of breast cancer and told me his plan was to give me four very aggressive rounds of chemo, then eight more that wouldn't be quite as aggressive. He told me I would lose my hair in a few weeks, that I would be fatigued and probably have some days when I would be very sick. I would come over the following Monday and start chemo. Then I would have a week off, then come over for lab work and then start over again. If my lab work showed my blood count was down, I would have to postpone the treatment until my blood count came back up. The nurses gave me a lot of literature to read that would explain about my treatments and all the side effects.

I left the office determined I would do what the doctors told me and trust in God to help me through what lay ahead. I had heard a lot of horror stories over the years about cancer and chemo and most of them were not good, but I knew everyone is different and I was determined I would make it with God's help. My doctor had given me the name of a place in Salem, Virginia where I could go and be fitted for a wig and prosthesis. I had decided again reconstruction surgery because the doctor had to cut so deep into my chest, I didn't know if the skin could be stretched enough to do any reconstruction. Also, I didn't want to face any more surgery and I knew I had a loving husband that didn't care one way or the other what my decision would be. I called the beauty shop, which was called Lorine's and made an appointment.

My first visit to Lorine's, I was still a little sore from my surgery. My sister, Joyce, went with me and when we met Lorine, I liked her from the start. She was an older lady and she had been battling cancer for years. Her cancer had affected her face and ear and she had had many surgeries, but she was a beautiful lady inside and out. Since I had already started my chemo and knew I would be losing my hair soon, I had her to fit me with a wig so I would be prepared when my hair came out. I had cut my hair short and Joyce had cut hers too to make me feel better. They fitted me with a wig close to the color and style of my own hair. They also fitted me for my prosthesis and my insurance paid for most of it along with some new bras.

The next trip I went to Lorine's, I was wearing my wig and most of my hair was gone. I had my wig styled and cut and she asked me if I wanted my hair buzzed. She said it didn't cost anything. I wasn't concerned about the cost. I didn't take time to think about it. I told her to go ahead and shave my head. As I looked into the mirror and saw what was left of my hair, it was much more traumatic than I thought it would be. My friend, Madeline was with me and I held back the tears. They would come later. After they put my wig back on, I felt a little better. I stopped at a beauty supply house on the way home and bought some turbans, some little skullcaps to wear around the house and one to sleep in. I silently wondered how long it would be before my hair would come back. I knew I had to take the good with the bad and I had to accept losing my hair and chemo and radiation treatments and whatever it took to help me get better. At least I had choices. Some people are given a diagnosis and it is too late to treat them.

In time, I would be glad I had my head shaved and got my wig because eventually, I was almost completely bald. The term "bald is beautiful" is not always true. I also lost my eyebrows and eyelashes. I also lost the hair under my arms and on my legs and believe it or not, it has never come back. This has been a blessing in disguise.

I would go to the doctor in between treatments and have lab work done. If my blood count was low, I had to have a shot in my upper arm. Sometimes I would have to have two. One was for the white count and one was for the red. These shots helped to bring up my blood count in order to take my chemo the next week. The shots were painful and I probably had about thirty-six during the time I was taking chemo. I was lucky in a way because my blood count never got so low that I had to skip a treatment. I tolerated the chemo quite well, although I did have days that I was very sick and weak. They gave me pills to take for the nausea and vomiting.

I started feeling a little better during my last treatments, so I decided to try to go back to work for a while and then work on my retirement. I called medical and set up an appointment. I had to be cleared before I could return to work. Everyone at medical was glad to see me and they asked me if I was sure I was ready to return to work. They also told me if I needed to come over anytime during work hours if I got sick or really tired not to hesitate to do so. Everyone thought I was crazy to return to work so soon, but at the time we only had my sick pay coming in. I wasn't making as much as I made working and my husband's disability check only came once a month. (He had so many health problems that he had gotten disability from social security. He would later get complete disability from the government because of Agent Orange and the time he had spent in Vietnam.) I had to at least go back to work and try it. I knew if it got too hard, I could work out on sick leave again.

Soon it was time for me to go and take my first chemo treatment. My husband went with me. On the way over, I was dreading it because I didn't know what to expect. When we got to the office, they checked my blood pressure and temperature and led me back to a room that was filled with chairs that looked somewhat like recliners. Most of them were occupied and I would learn as the months went by, that you usually just took the first available one and in some cases have to wait until there was one available.

As I sat down, the nurse asked me if I wanted a snack. I told her no. She got me a pillow for my neck and a blanket. There were magazines and books to read and a television. Some people were reading, some were watching television and some were sleeping. Soon they hooked me up to an i.v. This contained medicine to keep me from getting sick. After this was administered, they hooked me up to the chemo. The chemo was a dark orange and I learned later it was called "Red Devil." It was one of the most powerful chemos and it was very aggressive. It kills all the cells in your body, including the good ones. The good ones replenish themselves, but in some cases, some people have to have bone marrow transplants.

The whole procedure took about an hour and soon they unhooked me and told me they would see me in two weeks. My husband was in the waiting room and I told him I was ready to go. We went out to eat, but I couldn't eat very much. I would learn as the months went by how the chemo takes your appetite and nothing tastes quite right. Some people describe it as a metallic taste in your mouth. I would learn that on good days, when my food tasted somewhat normal, I would take advantage and eat some of the good things I liked.

I would have four strong treatments and then eight not so strong. I would lose my hair in a few weeks. It would come out in my hands in clumps when I shampooed my hair or I would find it on my pillow.

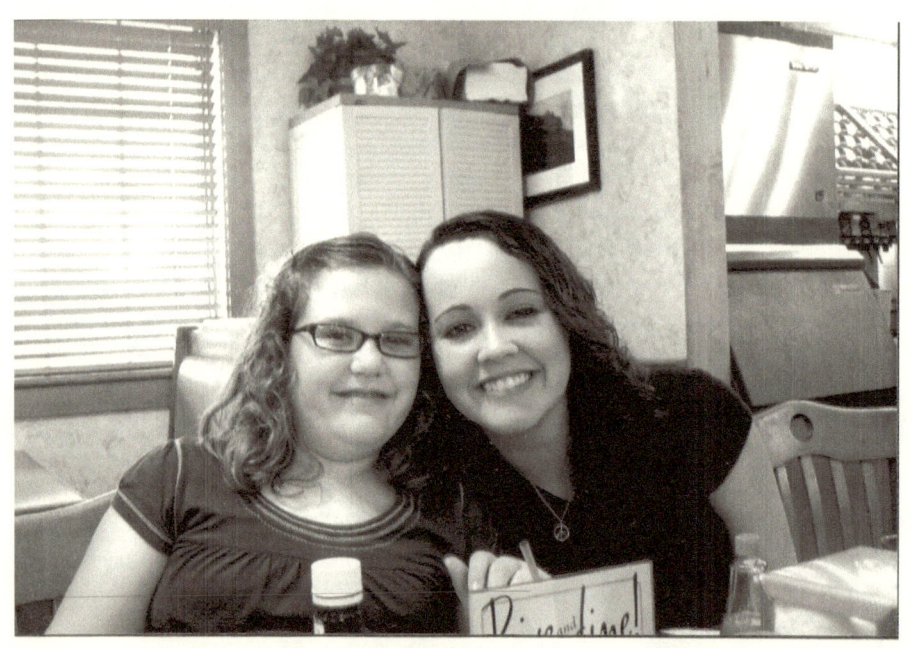

Laney and Sydney, Ryan's—2010.

Chapter IX

"Another Detour"

I had been off for five months. It was January, 2004. It seemed strange going through the gate at work. As I climbed the steps and started seeing some of my friends, they would approach me and hug me and tell me how good I looked. I went to my locker and got my "tools" and went out onto the floor where I worked. On my job, we needed to relieve the person going off on the shift before us. I saw Jerry, a friend of mine, coming toward me with a smile. He hugged me and said, "Eleanor, you look so good, you have a glow about you." I told him it wasn't me, but the one who lived inside of me and who had brought me this far.

After a few weeks back at work, I soon settled into the old routine. I had so much support from my co-workers and my bosses. I would get a little tired, but all in all I did o.k. I was still finishing up my chemo treatments, but I tried to use my vacation days when I had a treatment scheduled.

In March, we had a trip scheduled to go to North Carolina. I was one of the safety captains and each year, we would visit our customers. It was called a safety share and we had a good relationship with them. My friends begged me to go one last time and I decided I would. We would usually go down and spend the night and come back the next day. We would meet at the gatehouse on the 24th, drive down and return on the 25th. We usually rode down in company cars or sometimes we rented a van. We always had fun on the way down and we usually stopped somewhere for breakfast.

We arrived at the plant around noon. We stopped and got our passes and a guide would take us to a meeting room. We went to the ladies room to freshen up and we had to step up into the restroom. I made the comment that they should have a sign there that would tell people to watch their step. We decided when we did our safety audit, we would mention this. After we freshened up, we returned to the meeting room and we mingled with everyone and then had lunch brought in and we ate as we conducted the meeting.

After the meeting, we went to the restroom again. We were getting ready to go on a tour of the plant and do a safety check. As I was coming out of the restroom, I forgot about the step, missed it as I stepped forward and down I went. I fell hard on my left side. As I slid across the floor, I felt a sharp pain shoot through my shoulder. I also hit my head on a table that was right outside the restroom. Thank God, my wig cushioned the blow to my head.

Everyone gathered around me and one of my friends went to get the plant nurse. When they came back, I heard the nurse tell them to sit me up. As they did, I felt myself pass out from the pain. The next thing I remember, they were loading me onto a stretcher, putting me into an ambulance, and taking me to the nearest hospital. I felt so strange. By the time I got to the hospital, my senses had returned. I felt so bad because I believed that this would really put a damper on the trip. I also felt foolish for falling and getting hurt, especially on a safety trip.

After they x-rayed my shoulder and head, it turned out my head was alright, but my shoulder was broken. I had suspected this because of the pain. They gave me a morphine shot for the pain and a nice elderly black gentlemen came in and put my arm in a sling. After a while we all returned to the motel where we were staying. I decided I would stay the night and return home in the morning. I did have my friends to call my family and tell them what happened so they wouldn't be too surprised when I came home.

My friend, Pat, made sure I took my medicine during the night. All the others went out to eat and I begged her to go, but she insisted on staying with me and keeping an eye on me. All the others came by when they came back to see how I was doing. I sat up in bed propped up with pillows and tried to doze a little. The next morning, we returned home in the company car and I had to go by our plant so they could do an accident investigation. Of course, the news had already gotten back to the plant about my accident. We met at the gatehouse and discussed exactly how my accident had happened, then I had to see the plant doctor. He told me I would be off from work a while and he sent me to an orthopedic surgeon.

The day I went to see the surgeon, they x-rayed my shoulder. As I went in to see the doctor, he told me it was a "clean" break and I wouldn't have to have surgery. I breathed a sigh of relief. However, he told me I would have to have several weeks of physical therapy and that it would be about a year before my arm would heal properly.

The therapy was rough. Sometimes I felt they were pulling my arm out of the socket. I also had exercises to do at home. Eventually, I finished the therapy and I can honestly say my shoulder healed wonderfully and it only hurts a little once in a while when the weather is bad.

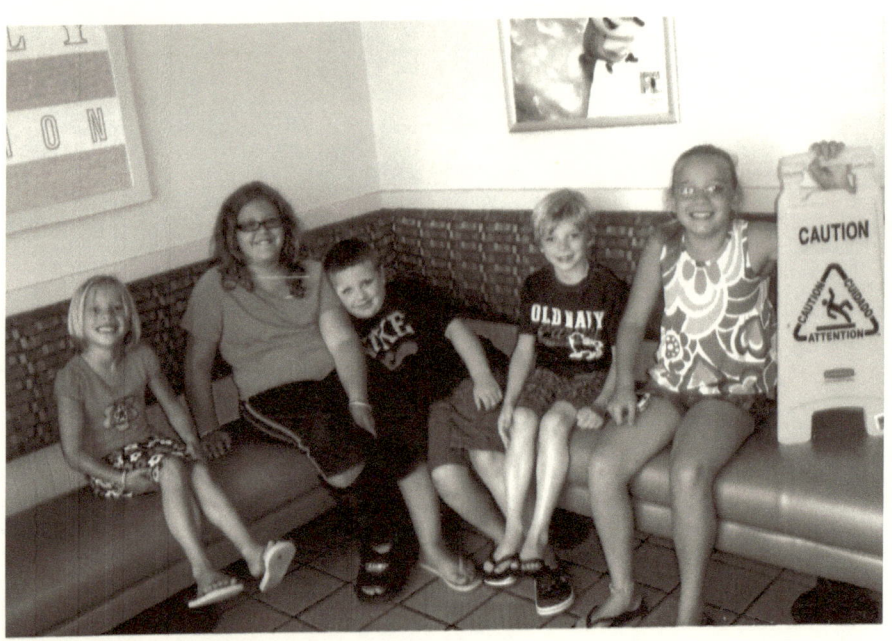

Zoe, Cameron, Ryan, Brennen and Laney—IHOP 2010.

CHAPTER X

"Radiation Therapy"

With God's help I made it through all the chemo and went back to the doctor to set up my radiation. My hair started growing back during my last treatments, and it was very curly. I was so glad to have some, I didn't care if it was straight or curly, red or green. As it began to grow back, I wore a hat for a while, and then although it was very short, I went without the hat. Most of my friends knew why my hair looked like it did, anyway.

I would take my radiation treatments in a different hospital than my chemo treatments. I would go to Pulaski, Virginia for my radiation. I had to travel about thirty miles of so, but that wasn't so bad. I had to go Monday through Friday and off on week-ends. They try to schedule you for the same time every day, but because I worked shift work, they had to adjust to my schedule.

When I met my radiation doctor, I liked her as soon as I set eyes on her. She was a beautiful black woman, impeccably dressed with a beautiful smile. Her name was Dr. Ojomo. She explained to me that I would have thirty-six treatments. The first day I would be tattooed and measurements taken. This would give them a field to work with to make sure the radiation would go exactly where it was supposed to.

The tattoos were really small. All of this took about an hour and soon I was done. I then set up my schedule to come for my treatments. I would come each morning except when I was on the daylight shift. Then I would come in the evenings.

I would go check in and wait in the waiting room until they called me. The waiting room had puzzles to work, a television, magazines and snacks. I met many people during the course of my treatments and many were a lot worse than me. Some had lost limbs, some were in wheelchairs and some were on oxygen twenty-four hours a day. Some were wearing implants that were injecting chemo into their bodies even as they were taking radiation. I learned to be thankful that I looked and felt better than most of them. Some had to travel a long way to get their treatments. The hospital offered transportation to those who couldn't afford the trip. I was so glad I didn't have far to travel. Most of the time my sister or my husband came with me. Sometimes I came by myself. I would learn the worst side effect of radiation is the tiredness.

As my treatments progressed, I would go check in and they would send me on in to put my gown on and wait in the hall outside the treatment room. Most of the time things went pretty fast. Once in a while, they would be behind or the machine would be down. They only had one when I started, but they later got a second one which helped speed things up a lot.

The treatment room was very cold. You had to remove your gown and you would feel exposed. Sometimes I would have young interns and some of them were males younger than my sons. I felt a little embarrassed, but soon I learned to take it all in stride and know they were only there to learn and do their jobs. I usually had the same nurses and they were always nice and courteous and we often talked about our families and other things to get our mind off the treatment.

A few days before I started my treatments, my daughter-in-law, Hilary, had called me and told me she had a dream that I was laying on a table taking my treatments and there were angels around me. I remembered this as I progressed into my treatments and I would try to envision this and I really could see angels in my mind, but they were usually in the form of Della Reese or Romey Downey. I would also imagine the radiation zapping the cancer from my body.

There was a big control room the technician would go into before I started the treatment. They could see me at all times and I had to lie perfectly still. They would tell you when they were about to turn on the machine. It was very loud and menacing, but painless. The treatment didn't take long, but on some of the days they had to do X-rays and it took a little longer. I would see the doctor once a week and she would check on my progress.

After each treatment, I would count down-30 more, 29 more and eventually I knew it would all be finished. The treatments did burn my skin and they gave me cream to use, which helped. After about a week, the fatigue set in. They had told me this would happen and would probably last for a while even after I had completed the treatments.

During the course of my treatments, I faced another obstacle. As I told you, we had to see the doctor once a week and I had thought I felt a small lump in my right breast. I told Dr. Ojomo about it and when she examined me, it was very tender. She decided I should have a mammogram. I had one when my cancer was discovered the first time, but I only had it on my left breast because we all focused on it.

I did go and have another mammogram and ultrasound and the results were not good, so they wanted me to have another biopsy. I had this in October, 2004 and after waiting for a week or so, my surgeon called and told me he needed to see me. I knew something was up or he would have given me the results over the phone. After I went to see him, it seemed the cancer had returned in my right breast. It was a little over a year since my cancer had been discovered and now the same kind was in my right breast.

It was really hard to hear this, I think even harder than the original diagnosis. I was now facing another mastectomy, chemo and possibly radiation again. The hardest part of my battle was having to tell my family my cancer had returned and I hated seeing the concerned looks on their faces. It was also difficult not seeing the grandkids as much as I wanted. I had to miss so much with them when I was taking chemo because I had to be so careful not to be around anyone sick because of my immune system. I had already missed one year of my life taking treatments and being sick and now I was facing another.

All my sisters were concerned for me, but my youngest sister, Joyce, was a rock for me during this time. She tended to look on the bright side of things and she told me I might not have to take chemo again. Of course, there were a lot of prayers going up for me. I think I was on every prayer list of every church around because of all my friends.

It was hard losing my right breast and again they took out lymph nodes and they were all malignant, too. I was very fortunate, though, because after I saw my oncologist again, he told me he would consult with Dr. Ojomo and see if I could take radiation again. It turned out that I could, and even though I wouldn't be taking chemo, I had to take hormones along with this.

I returned to my radiation doctor and she set me up for thirty more treatments on my right side. I continued to work for a while and sometimes I would work all day and go straight to my treatment. This took a toll on me and everyone couldn't believe I was working and going through treatments again. I knew my strength was coming from a higher power and that it wouldn't be too long until I could retire.

I had to change my retirement date because of being off with my shoulder. My retirement day did finally arrive. I went in on the 11-7 shift. They gave me a special breakfast and took up money for me. It's hard to explain sometimes how you feel when you leave a place you have worked at for 37 years. The people are like your second family. You know all about them and their families and they know all about you and yours. That last night was hard. I didn't have to do any work. They had someone in my place. I tried to go around the shop and see everyone. Good-byes have always been hard for me. I knew in my heart, that some of these people I would never see again, but I knew my close friends would stay in touch.

I not only went around and talked to the people, but I walked around and thought of all the memories over the years. About five a.m., I went to the locker room, just to look around and reminisce. I had already cleaned my locker out and had taken most of my things home the week before. About 5:30 a.m., I decided I would try to slip out quietly for the last time. I went downstairs and started out the door and a couple of people saw me and had to come and give me one more hug. The walk from the building to the gatehouse that I had walked so many times seemed like a mile that morning. I finally went through the gate, dropped off my badge at the gatehouse and headed to my car. As I walked through the parking lot, little did I know what lie ahead for me.

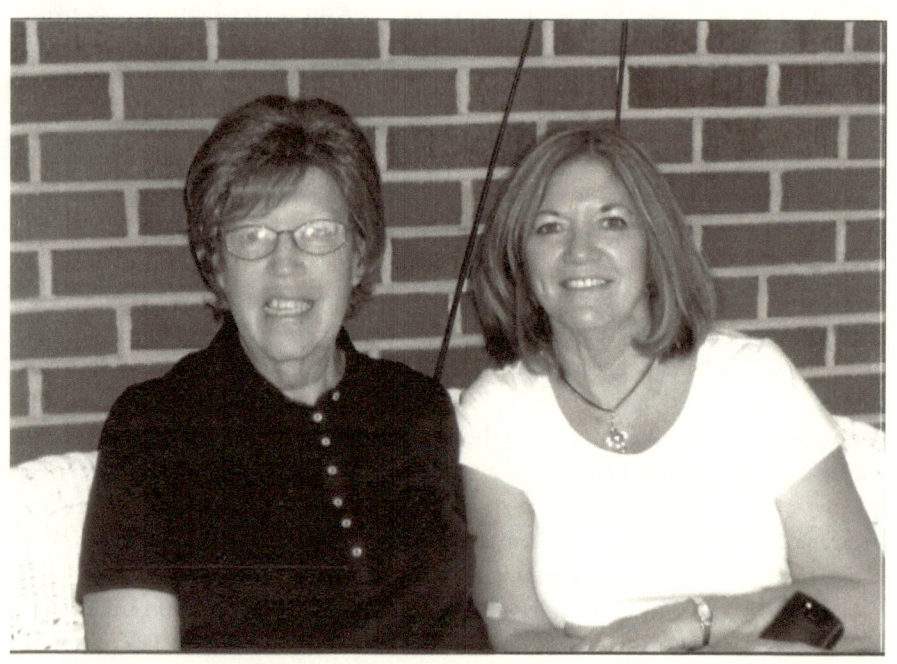

Me and Joyce at my sister Hazel's house, 2010.

Chapter XI

"Another Unexpected Diagnosis"

I had a friend, Carol, who was diagnosed with the same kind of cancer as mine. We often talked on the phone and I remember her telling me in one of our conversations that she had some little red places come up in her chest area. In the back of my mind, I remembered reading on the internet about our type of breast cancer and how it could show up in the form of little bumps that look like mosquito bites. It is not skin cancer, but it is sometimes associated with inflammatory breast cancer. Soon after she told me about these bumps, she called me after returning to her doctor and sure enough, it was cancer again. I tried to reassure her, but I felt so bad that her cancer had come back. She had just recently retired too.

I have had bad knees for quite a while. I suffered from osteoarthritis in both my knees. Over the years, I had injections of cortisone, laparoscopic surgery in my right knee not to mention all the pain medication I had taken over the years. My left knee got so bad I decided to have knee replacement I had friends who had had this done and it seemed to help them with the pain and mobility. I had it done as an outpatient in May of 2005. I got through the surgery, but the doctor put me on Coumadin, which is a blood thinner to prevent blood clots. I had to have my blood checked often and I began to feel really tired and run-down. I spent a lot of time on the couch and everyone told me how bad I looked. One Friday, they called me from the hospital and told me it was critical I get there as soon as possible. They asked me if I had been bleeding anywhere (I hadn't), and they told me I could be bleeding internally. My husband took me to the hospital and we went straight to the emergency room. They gave me a shot of Vitamin K and I started feeling better in a few days and was able to come off the Coumadin.

After about a week, I started physical therapy on my knee. I was glad I got to see all of my friends at the hospital again, but the therapy was very painful. I would go two or three times a week and also do some of the exercises at home. Each time I returned to my doctor, they would send a report on my progress.

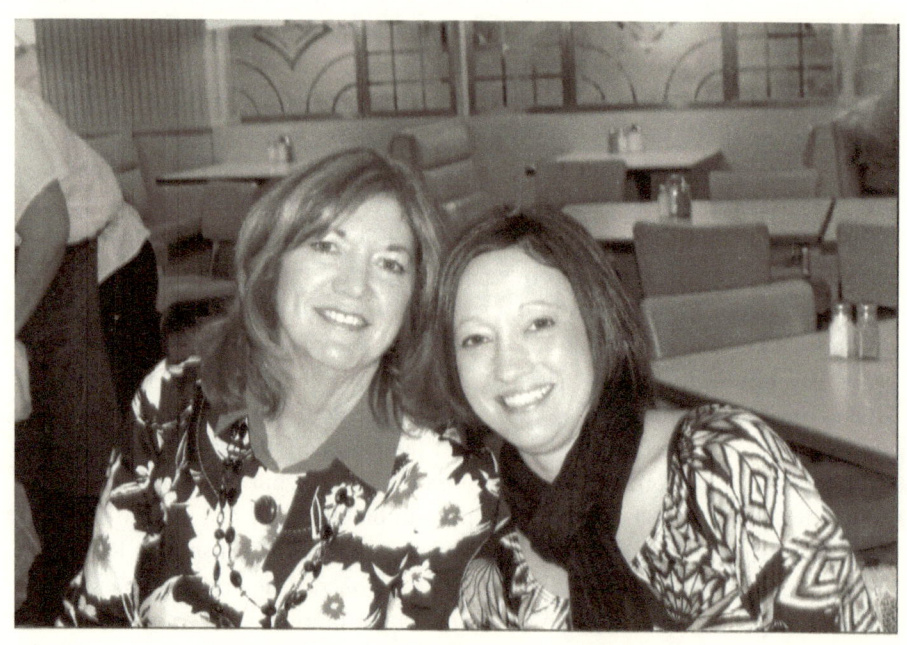

My sister Joyce and Angie, Travis' sister.

Chapter XII

"Here We Go Again"

During this time, one day I got out of the shower and noticed some little red bumps on my chest. My first thought was that these were the same ones Carol had told me about. I thought they might be from the Coumadin. When I returned to my oncologist he was concerned. He sent me back to my surgeon to have another biopsy and he was also concerned. He took a sample of two of the bumps and sent them off. In a few days, he called me and sure enough, my cancer was back.

When I went back to Dr. McCoy, I asked him if I could have radiation again. He told me to check with my radiation doctor and after talking with her, I was set up for radiation again. This time I would have about thirty treatments. I continued to take physical therapy in addition to my radiation treatments.

With God's help, I finished all the radiation treatments and the physical therapy. My body was so tired and I asked God to please give me a little break. The radiation did take care of the cancer and I did get a break for a while. I enjoyed this time so much because I began to get some strength back and since I was retired now, I could take my time at home when I was doing laundry or housework. Some days, if I was tired, I waited until the next day to do some of my chores. I also spent as much time with my family and friends as I could. Some of the best times were birthday parties and cookouts or all of us going out to eat somewhere.

Things went along smoothly for a while. Then the bumps showed up on my right side. I thought "Oh, no, here we go again." This time when I saw Dr. McCoy, he didn't even have me do a biopsy. He and I both knew what it was. I took radiation again and he also put me on another hormone pill.

In the meantime, my friend, Carol seemed to get worse. She and I were having about the same treatments, except she had never taken radiation. Where my treatments seemed to be working, nothing they were doing for her seemed to help. She lost her battle and I was devastated. One of the hardest things for me other than having to tell my family each time my cancer returned was losing so many of my friends to this dreaded disease. Only someone who has experienced what we have can understand. We belong to an exclusive club that we wouldn't want anyone else to belong to. I know we are not supposed to question God, but sometimes I wondered why He takes some and leaves others. I know in my heart He left me for a purpose and I know one of those purposes it to get this book out to encourage other people who are going through this battle, too. I know God has used me a lot with my testimony, but I know this book can reach a lot more.

I have been singing all my life and I also play the keyboard and guitar. I have been singing in church for many years, but I had to give it up for a while because I just didn't have the strength. My music director and friend at church, Terri, told me to let her know when I felt like singing again and she would put me back on the schedule.

My niece had bought me a CD with a song on it called, "Just Another Hill." I was listening to it in the car one day and all I could do was cry. It sounded exactly like what I was going through. I knew I had to have the soundtrack. I finally found it one day. I decided to try to sing it at home. I have a den in the basement where I have my computer, my keyboard and a karaoke machine. The first time I tried to sing it, again all I could do was cry I wondered how I would ever be able to sing it in church.

I practiced it a few more times and I decided it was time. I told Terri she could put me back on the singing schedule. Of course, I was doing a lot of praying. When the night came for me to sing, I felt like I was singing in church for the first time. I gave my testimony before I sang because I promised God I would do this every chance I got. After the testimony, I sang and I just let God take control. I always pray that when I sing it will bless someone. I had several people come up to me after the service and tell me how the song had touched them. I knew it would be easier the next time. I am a firm believer that if you have gifts and talents, you should use them. I may not be the best singer in the world, but my heart is in the right place and I try to pick songs that will bless someone in a special way.

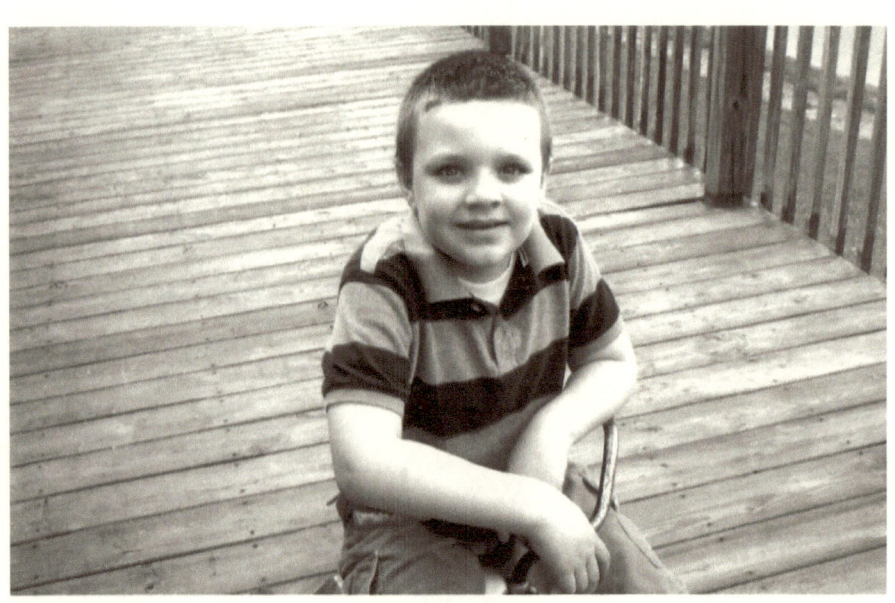

My "Little Man", Ryan Zane.

CHAPTER XIII

"Continuing The Battle"

During all my battles, I did a lot of praying and sometimes I would just ask God to give me a break. He always did, sometimes it was a short one and other times it was a little longer. During these times, I felt well and whole. I had more strength and I was able to do more, especially around the house. I continued to get tired from time to time, but I had learned to rest when I needed to. After all, most things could wait until another day. It was hard for me when I had to turn down babysitting for my grandkids. My kids never asked me too often, but when they did sometimes and I had to say no. They always understood.

Each time my cancer returned, they would try a different form of treatment. The third time I was put on a hormone called Femora It continued to work for a while. Then I was on a hormone shot. I took one of these once a month and they had to be injected into my hip and were rather painful. I was taking these and also taking radiation again. I would wind up taking radiation three different times. It really concerned me taking all this radiation, but I had trust in Dr. Ojomo and I knew if she thought it was too much, she would tell me.

During my fifth bout with cancer, I was put on a chemo pill called Xeloda. It worked for quite a while, but had many side effects. Sometimes you have diarrhea and vomiting. You never know when you are going to get sick. Sometimes I would plan on going out and I would get sick and have to cancel. These pills are very powerful. You take eight pills a day for fourteen days, then off for seven and then start the cycle all over again. They are not only powerful, but also very expensive. I am so thankful my insurance paid it all but fifty dollars each time I had to refill them.

One of the worst side effects I had is called hand and foot syndrome. Some of my friends who had been on Xeloda had told me about this. Sometimes you have swelling and tingling in your hands and feet, but the worst is that your skin gets so dry and it tends to get very sore and crack and peel. I had tried everything, including a medicine that was developed from a cream they use on horses. I have learned to control it pretty well. I am thankful because even with the side effects, it is better than taking full-blown chemo through your veins. I have been told by my oncologist that I would take this medicine as long as it was working. I know if it quit working, I would have to try something else. I also know that I will have to take some form of treatment for the rest of my life. I also know that is a small price to pay if it prolongs your life.

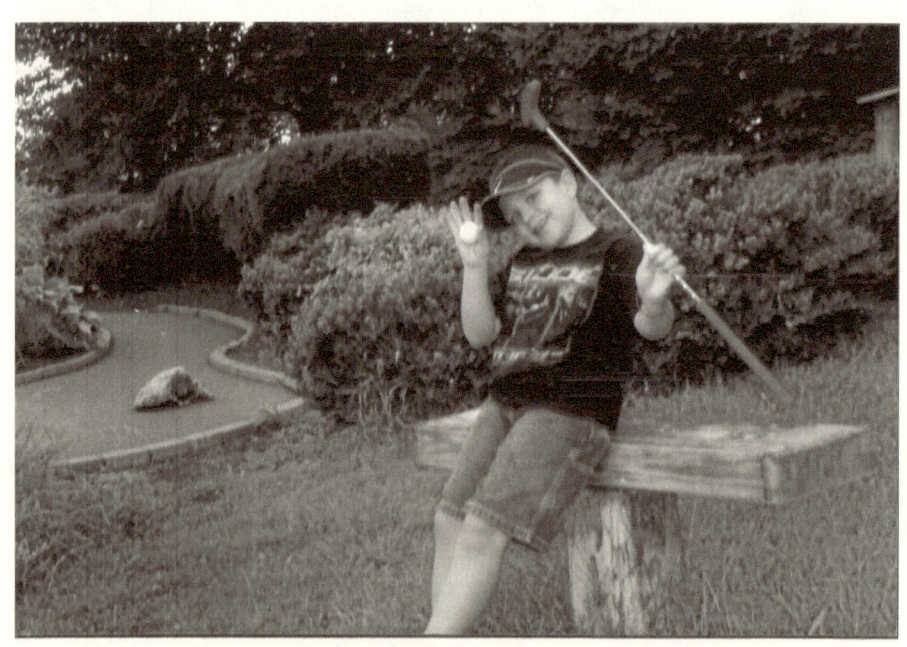

Ryan at Minature Golf, 2010.

CHAPTER XIV

"Proud Moments"

Some of my proudest moments have been when I was able to walk in Relay for Life. We have one in our hometown each year around June or July. I was unable to attend until 2005. I have tried to go every year since. It felt so good to make a lap or two around the field and look at all the faces that you know are survivors and going through the same things that you are. It is even more fulfilling to hear the cheers from the crowds that attend. Our county has been doing this for several years and they have raised a lot of money.

I was also privileged to attend the one at Virginia Tech a couple of times. Of course, I didn't know any of the people I walked with, but it didn't matter. We were all there for the same purpose. When you round the track, you can't explain to anyone else the feeling you get. My sister, Joyce, went with me to the ones at Tech. She worked there as a secretary for twenty-five years, so she knew her way around the campus. When I came around and met her at the end of the lap, I could see the tears in her eyes and of course, they were in mine too. I hope to be able to do it again.

As I write this book, it is nearing the end of April, 2007. I was invited again to walk in the Relay for Life at Tech. I had my sister to respond to the e-mail and let them know we would attend again. Little did we know before we were to go there on April 20th, the events that would take place.

On April 16, Joyce called me and asked me if I had been watching the news. I told her no. She said they were telling that there was an incident at Tech, possibly a shooting. I immediately turned on CNN and they were announcing that there indeed had been a shooting and a young girl and boy had been shot. The boy was a resident advisor and had supposedly broken up a domestic dispute and he and the girl were killed. They were questioning a suspect that they thought was her boyfriend. This was disturbing enough, but later in the day they announced there had been another shooting in Norris Hall and there were possibly 30 causalities. I immediately became numb and started crying and I, like so many others wondered what in the world was going on. I live in Pearisburg and we are about 30 or 40 minutes away from Tech. As I said, my sister had worked there for many years and even though she had retired, she went back from time to time to fill in when they needed her. I was so glad she wasn't there that day. Over the next hour or so, we all stayed glued to the television and called each other every few minutes.

As the story unfolded, it seemed a Korean student name Cho Seung-Hue was the shooter. He had waited almost two hours after killing the first two at West Amber, and then he went to Norris Hall and killed 30 people, some students and some professors and finally killed himself. He had chained the doors and by the time the police were alerted and gotten in, it was all over. There were also many wounded. This was called a massacre and was the worst school shooting in American history. It would affect not only the nation, but also the whole world. For a week or so, the nation mourned and everyone became a Hokie.

We weren't sure they would still have the relay only a few days after this tragedy, but they did and we decided to go. It was very moving and they dedicated a portion of it to the fallen heroes. News media were everywhere, but they weren't allowed on the field where we were walking our survivor lap. One of the students who was killed, a young girl, had raised the most money for the relay. We also lost one of our own, a young man from Narrows, Virginia, only 3 miles away. His name was Jarrett Lane and he was only a few months from graduation and had already been accepted at another school to further his education.

This was such a senseless tragedy and I know we as humans can't understand why things like this happen just as I wonder why I have gone through all I have. The old saying, "Bad things happen to good people" is true. We shouldn't ask, "Why me?", but we should ask "Why not me?" Why did a local family lose six of their nine children in a gas explosion in Michigan? Only a month ago, he blessed them with another precious baby, a little girl they named Markita Joelle. Markita means "Little Mark" after her dad and Joelle means "He is Lord."

I am always reminded there is good that comes from tragedy although we can't always see it at the time. I try to face each day and enjoy it. Even when I wake up and feel my aches and pains and stiffness, I get up and start facing another day after I have my morning coffee and try to make the most of each day. We never know when it might be our last. It might be the last time to tell someone we love them and we should do this each day. We should reach out and help everyone we can and not worry about our needs, but how we can help others. I once heard Oprah Winfrey say, "We get out of the world what we put into it." I have never forgotten this. If we put out negativity, that is what we get back. If we put out love, we get love back.

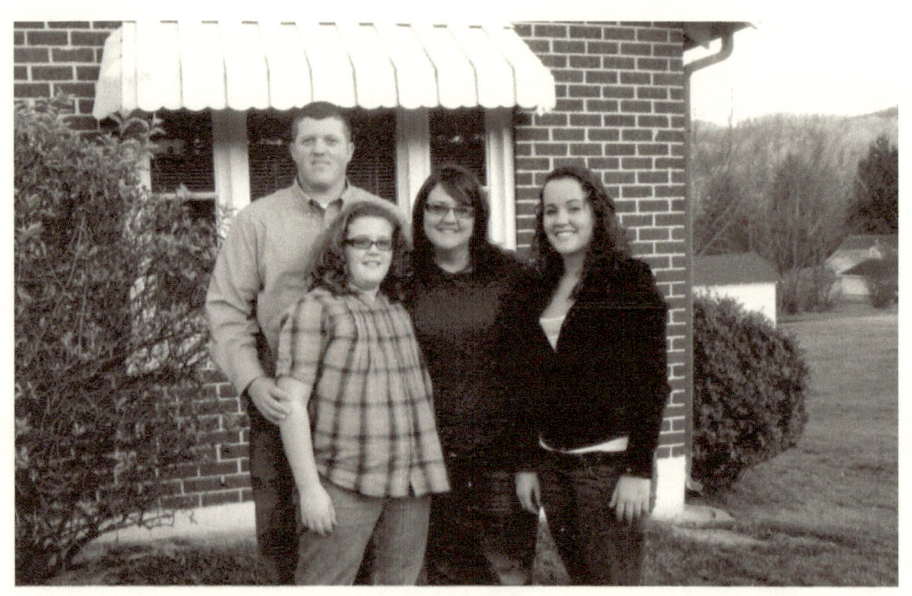

Rusty, Bridget, Sydney and Laney, Thanksgiving 2010.

CHAPTER XV

"God's Unseen Hand"

So many times in life, we take things for granted. It can be our family, our friends, our finances, our health. I look back on my life and God reminds me of all the times he has blessed me in all areas of my life. He also reminds me of the times He has had His hand on me when I did something stupid. A few years back, I had traveled to Pulaski, Virginia to visit my oldest sister who was in a rehab facility after suffering a stroke. She is now in a nursing home in Dublin, Virginia.

After visiting her at the rehab, I decided to go to a little drive-in called Sonic and get something to eat. It is one of my favorite places to eat. Not only is the food good, but it takes you back to times in the fifties and sixties like the movie "American Graffiti. They play old music over the intercom. You pull in, drive up to one of the stations, push a button, and order what you want. The waitresses bring your food out to the car; some of them even wear roller skates. This is one of the few places they still have curb service. I try to always give them a good tip because I remember many years ago when I worked at a similar place and you make more in tips than your paycheck.

On the way to Sonic, my mind wandered and I missed the turnoff I went on down another block or so and knew I could cut back to the left and still get to Sonic. It had been a while since I had been on this end of town, and I forgot they have some one-way streets. Yes, you guessed it, I turned down one. I realized this when I saw oncoming traffic. I was in the right lane, but so was another car coming my way. Thank goodness, they saw what I had done and gave me time to cut into a parking lot and turn around. I, of course, said a quick prayer of thanks. I told this in church later and told them if the Lord didn't look out for us, I would have been gone a long time ago.

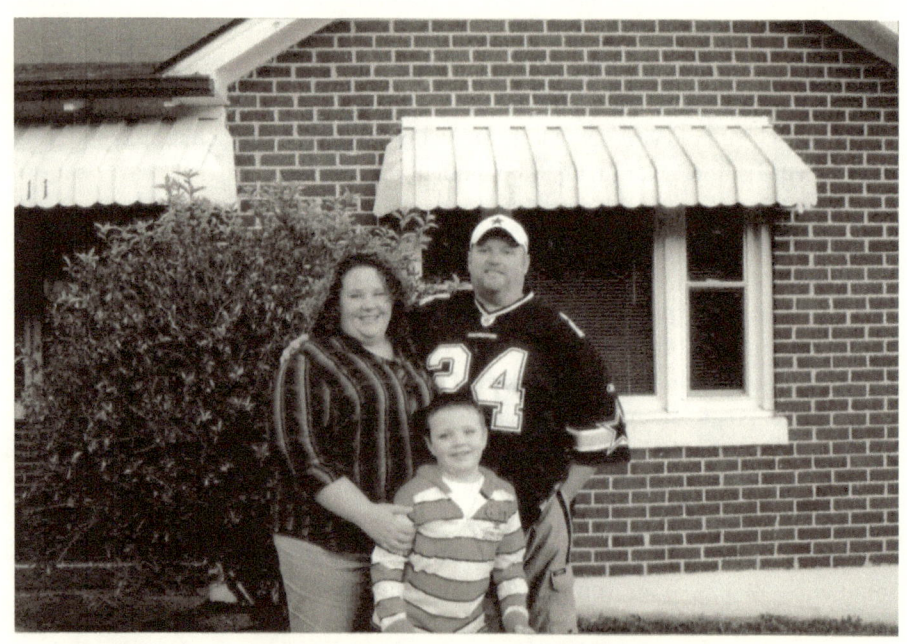

Hilary, Randy and Ryan, Thanksgiving 2010.

Chapter XVI

"Another Setback"

I had begun to have shortness of breath and my energy level was very low. I would get out of breath just walking from room to room. The smallest chore I did at home, I would be exhausted. I knew from talking to my radiation doctor that I would always have some shortness of breath because of all the radiation I had taken. Also, I had an appointment with my oncologist in a few days and I knew he would give me a good check-up.

The day of my doctor visit, I picked up my friend, Madeline, and I let her drive. As soon as she saw me and heard me talking almost in a whisper, she knew something was wrong. When I got to the doctor's office and he started checking me, I could see the concern on his face. He said he was afraid I had a blood clot in my lungs or that my cancer had returned. I didn't get scared because I decided a long time ago that I had put my faith in God and He is in control of my life and my health. Dr. McCoy sent me straight to the hospital to have a scan on my lungs.

When we got to the hospital, I checked in and waited for them to call me back to the lab. I went to the bathroom and while I was in there, I prayed. Again, I wasn't afraid. I just asked God to help me accept whatever the test results would show. We went to the lab and I didn't have to wait too long until they came and got me for my scan. The nurse had to put an I.V. into my vein in my arm. I told her how hard it was to find my veins. After much probing, she eventually inserted the needle. I have been stuck so many times over the years; this is just another thing I tolerate. The scan only took a few minutes. She told me they would call my doctor and he would call me with the results.

We decided to go get something to eat while we waited on the call from the doctor. We went to IHOP which was close to the hospital. After what seemed like an eternity, Dr. McCoy called and told me they had found something in the upper lobe of one of my lungs, but he thought it was an infection and he was going to call me in an antibiotic. He also told me he wanted to see me in a week.

After I got back home, I went and picked up my prescription and started taking it right away. After a few days, I started to feel a little better although my arm was black and blue where the needle had been inserted. When I returned the next week to see Dr. McCoy, he told me that I had pneumonia. He was really relieved that I didn't have a blood clot. So was I. I had never had pneumonia before, but I knew it was better than a blood clot. Eventually, my strength began to return and I was able to get back to my regular activities.

As I told you, it seems when something happens to me, something happens to my husband. He had a place on his lip that wouldn't heal. We kept telling him to go have it checked. He also had a place on his neck and on his arm. We were more concerned about his lip. Although he had given up smoking years ago, he still chewed. Although I hated the habit, I tried not to make a big deal about it because I was afraid he would start smoking again.

He finally went to see our family doctor and he sent him to a specialist. After doing a biopsy on all three areas, he told him he would call and give him the results in a few days. A few days later, the call came. I answered the phone and I could tell on my caller ID that it was the doctor's office. I called to my husband, who was in the bedroom, but I listened in to hear the results. The two places on his arm and neck were superficial and could be treated with an ointment they prescribed. However, the one on his lip was skin cancer and they would call back and tell him when he could come in and have it removed. I was concerned, but I knew this doctor was a good doctor and plastic surgeon. Several of my friends had gone to him and had good results. Eventually, Roy went and had it removed and skin grafted and everything turned out fine.

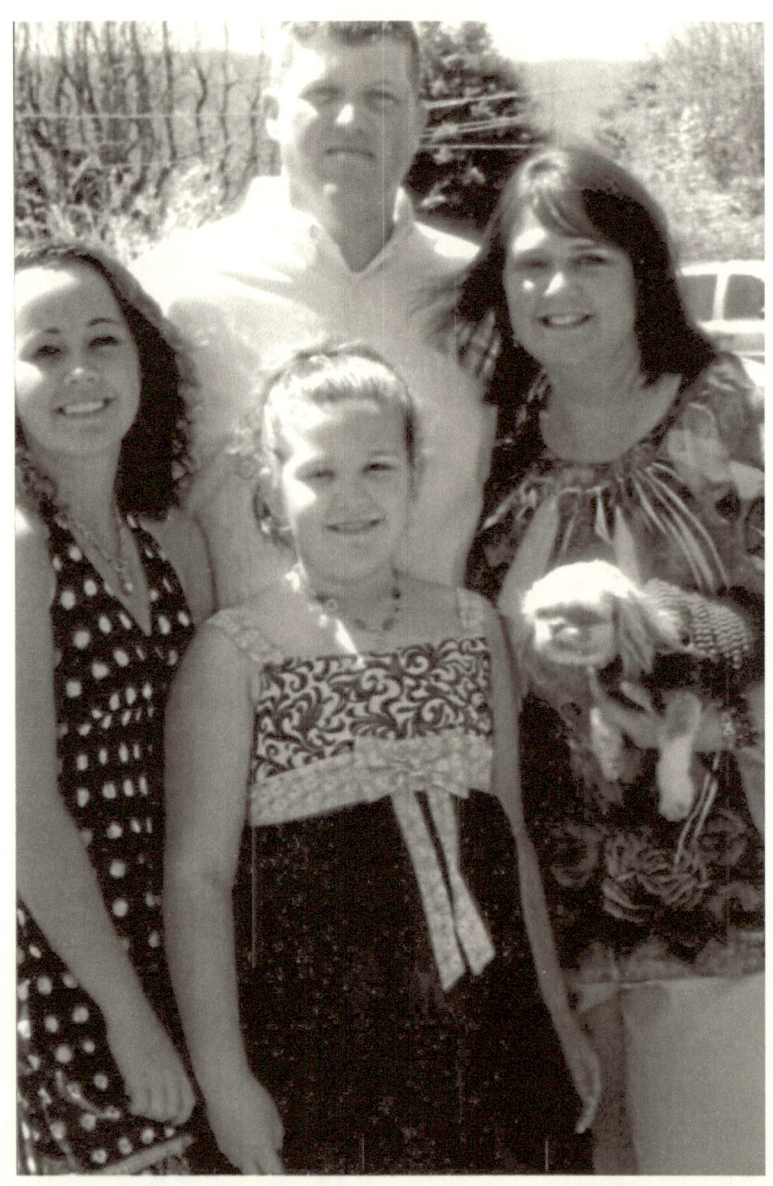

Rusty, Sydney, Bridget, Laney and "Izzy"—2010.

Chapter XVII

"Getting Used to Retirement"

It took some time for me to get used to having my husband home all the time and after I retired, it certainly took time for me to get used to not working. It has been over two years now since my retirement and my first battle with cancer.

I try to enjoy each day to the fullest. Sometimes we get up and my husband asks what's on the agenda for the day. Some days I have planned in advance and some days we just stay at home and work on things at home or just relax. I do a lot of crafts and my husband likes to work on lawnmowers and talk on the CB with his buddies. His handle is "Scooby Doo."

We have no promise of tomorrow and there is not a week goes by that it seems another of my friends pass away. Some of them I don't even know about until I read the obituaries. Some die from cancer, some from heart attacks, some from car wrecks or other accidents. I know I can count a lot of people that I used to work with that are gone now and some were only in their forties. I know who holds tomorrow and I know who holds my hand and until my time comes, I plan to make the most of my life and do all I can to help others along the way.

My mind goes back to one Christmas Eve when I was still working. I was on second shift which is 3-11. While most families were celebrating or getting ready to celebrate with their families and friends, I had to work. The factory where I worked operated twenty-four hours a day around the clock, year round. If you were scheduled to work, you worked or suffered the consequences. We were allowed to trade shifts with each other, but most people don't want the second shift on Christmas Eve.

Even though my family had already gotten together that morning to eat and open presents, I still felt a little sad to have to work. My family always celebrated on Christmas Eve, then we went to Roy's family on Christmas Day. It sure was a joy to see our grandchildren open their presents. Just to see their wide eyes and hear their glee as they tore into their presents was the best gift any grandparent could want.

Even though the last two months had been hard on me, I had a lot to be thankful for. I lost my precious mother on Nov. 30th, right after Thanksgiving. A few days after her death, my husband had a blocked carotid artery and had to have surgery. He was in the hospital for a week, but thankfully he got to come home before Christmas.

God reminds us that we have a lot to be thankful for even if we do have to work on Christmas. As I went to work that day, I reminded myself of all my wonderful blessings.

As I arrived at work and went to relieve the person going off, we exchanged greetings and wished each other a Merry Christmas. After I checked out my area I noticed a guy coming through on the trash route, a guy I had never seen before. This wasn't unusual because they were always sending people into different areas when they were short of labor, especially on holidays.

He approached me with a smile and said, "Just tell me, I'm doing a good job." I did and he laughed and told me he had never been in this area before and didn't even know where all the trash cans were.

I told him I would show him around and point out where all the trash cans were. As I did this, he began to tell me about himself. He had moved to our area from Las Vegas and his wife had recently died. He told me had prayed he wouldn't have to spend Christmas Eve alone, so when this job came up, he volunteered to work overtime.

I wished him a Merry Christmas and he went on his way. I thought "How Sad!" Even though I knew I might never see him again, I knew that sometimes God puts people in our paths at the right time. As the Bible says, "Sometimes we entertain angels unaware." I said a silent prayer for this stranger and as I went back to work, once again I thanked God for my blessings even though I was working on Christmas Eve.

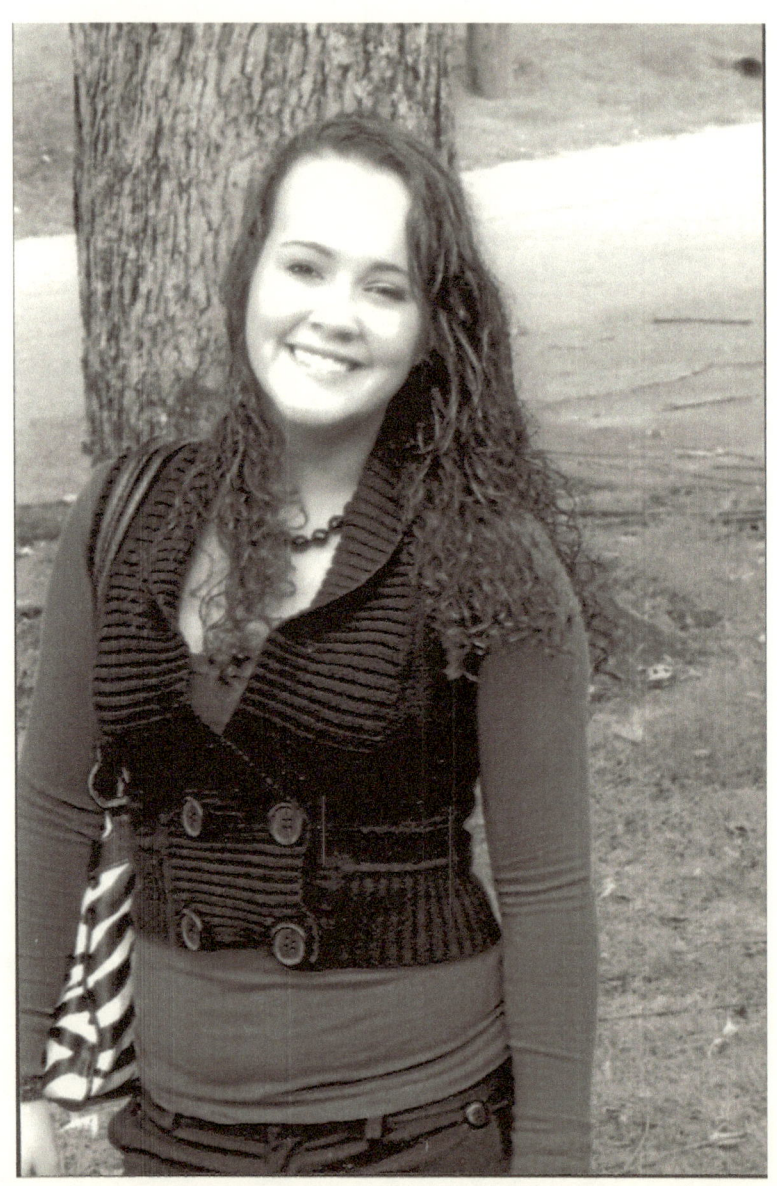

Sydney "Sweet Sixteen"—2010.

Chapter XVIII

"Remembering The Past"

I had a friend to tell me one time that the older we get, the more our mind wanders back to the past. I really believe this. Sometimes I'm just riding down the road and a memory will come to me. I think God reminds us of the plan He has for our life and how He has been putting it in place all our life. We don't always follow His plan, but He tries to keep us on course.

Several years ago at work, they told us they were going to offer college classes on site. They would bring in teachers and we could sign up for one class or several. They would pay for everything, including our books. The only thing was that the class had to be work related and help us on our jobs. I had always wanted to take a computer class, so I signed up.

The first day of class I was a little nervous. I knew all of my classmates because I worked with most of them or had at some point. Our teacher was a black lady from New River Community College and I liked her from the beginning. She made us feel so comfortable and I enjoyed the class so much, I kept taking more. Eventually I worked towards a goal. I obtained a certificate as an Administrative Assistant. I had to take some of my classes on line, but it wasn't long before I graduated with honors. My husband and my sister, Joyce, and my son and girlfriend at the time came, and I felt so proud that I was able to go back to school after all these years and accomplish this. This all happened before I got sick. My plans were to retire early and obtain a part-time job with the skills I now had. Our plans are not always God's plans, but I never regretted taking the classes They helped me a lot on my job and I just had the satisfaction of knowing you can still learn later in life and work towards a goal.

I was at a ladies meeting at church a couple of weeks ago and we were taking prayer requests. It dawned on me that 2007 was the first year since my first bout with cancer had been diagnosed that I hadn't had to have any treatments or tests. Other than my usual sickness from my pills and a bout with pneumonia, I had had a good year. This was really a blessing!

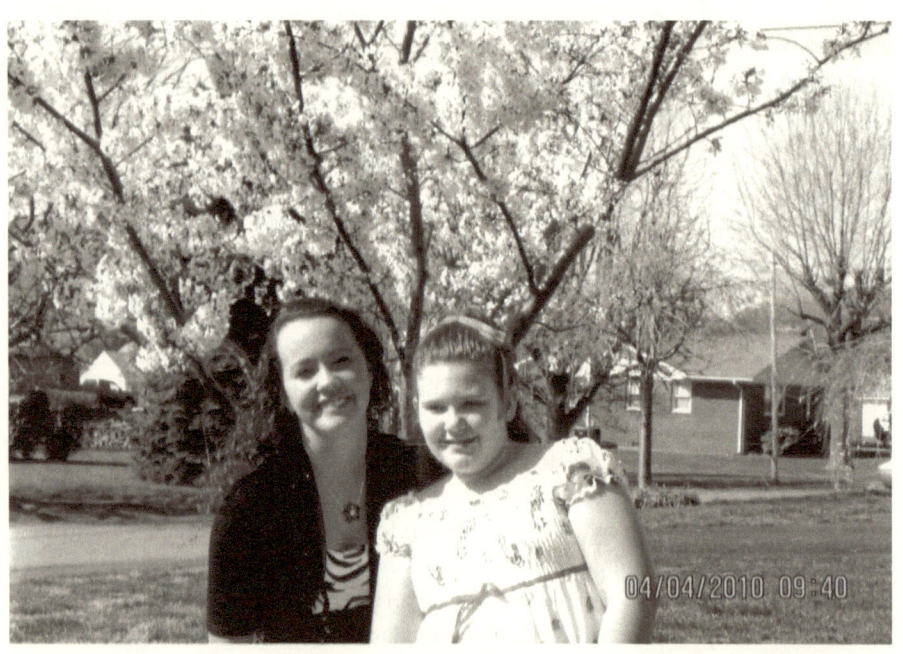

Sydney and Laney, Easter 2010.

Chapter XIX

"Another Knee Replacement"

It is now 2008 and we are halfway through the year. I turned 62 in May. At the beginning of May, I decided to have another knee replacement on my right knee. The pain had gotten so bad, I knew it was time. I had it scoped out about ten years ago, but it was getting worse and worse. Not only did I have pain, but I had trouble walking and especially going up and down steps. Since I seemed to be doing alright with my cancer, I decided now was as good a time as any while I had the nerve to do it. Some people, when they have one done, never do the other. That is also the reason some have both done at the same time. The surgeon who had done my left knee had moved away, so I asked Dr. McCoy if he could recommend someone. He told me about a Dr. LeBolt who some of his patients had used and they all liked him a lot. That was good enough for me. This time instead of ten minutes, I decided to do the shot. I took these home with me and I had to inject one into my stomach each day. These were to prevent blood clots. They weren't as painful as they sound and they were better than the coumadin.

After I called and made the appointment, I had to go to the hospital and have x-rays which they would send to Dr. LeBolt, prior to my appointment, which was over a month away. I wanted to have the surgery during the summer months, so I could get outside and walk and also so I wouldn't have problems with the weather when I went back for physical therapy.

The day of my appointment, I met the doctor and also his assistant, Beth. They were both really nice. They showed me my x-rays and I could see my knee was really bad. They told me I also had bone spurs behind my knee cap and the cartilage was completely worn out. They also told me there would be a lot of pain after the surgery because they would have to do a lot of cutting. I thought, "Oh, well, after all I have been through, I should be able to tolerate the pain. Boy, was I in for a rude awakening!

The day of my surgery came around and my husband and I made another trip to the hospital. We stopped and picked up my sister. Bless her heart! With all she had on her schedule, she still always took time to be with me when I needed her. It gave me great comfort.

My favorite part of surgery, if there is such a thing, is after you have been put to sleep and you start waking up, you know the surgery is over. You might be in pain and a little groggy, but at least you know it is over. One of my least favorite parts is that I always get so sick afterwards. Even when they add medicine to my i.v. to prevent nausea, I still get deathly sick. You mostly have the dry heaves, because there is nothing in your stomach to come up. I stayed two nights in the hospital and then I was able to go home. I never used a walker. I used a cane. When we got home, boy was I glad we had built a ramp going onto our deck that led into the front part of the house. We had done this before my first knee surgery and it was really a lifesaver. We had also had a walk-in shower installed and bars to hold on to. I was prepared this time. Roy had to practically carry me into the house the other time.

The first couple of weeks were so painful. I had pain medication and I used ice on my knee, but the pain was worse than any I had ever had including my two mastectomies. Sometimes I would cry. Roy would come walking through the hall, and tears would be running down my cheeks. He felt so helpless and said he didn't know what to do. I told him there was nothing he could do.

I started physical therapy and it was really hard, but I knew I had to work through the pain in order to get better. I did enjoy seeing my physical therapists again and catching up on things. They were all so good to me and I often took them goodies.

Dr. LeBolt had told me that after about two months, I wouldn't regret the surgery. Well, it took me a little longer, but one day I realized I didn't have pain any more. I have never regretted I had it done. I can get out and walk now, which I love to do and most important of all, I can get up off chairs and couches without help.

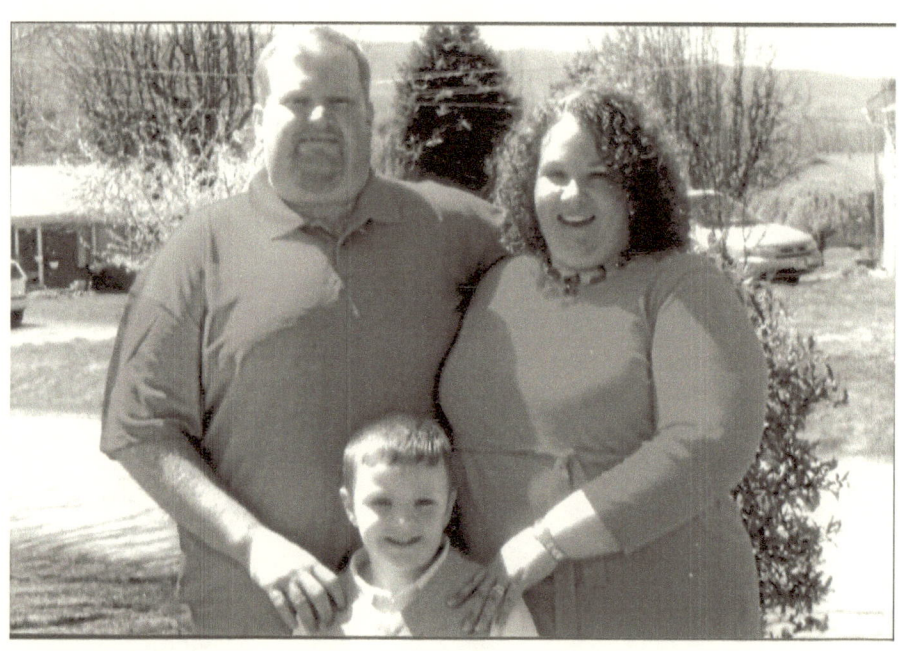

Randy, Hilary and Ryan, Easter 2010.

Chapter XX

"Another Setback"

As I finish this book, I am going through yet another battle. In the last couple months, my back had started hurting. I thought it was lower back pain. I even made an appointment with my chiropractor. I had gone to him for years when I was experiencing back problems, and he had helped me, so I decided it was worth a try. It was good to see him again and after about three treatments, my back pain seemed to be getting worse, so I told him I wanted to stop the treatments until I had seen my oncologist for my check-up. He agreed.

After I went for my check-up, I told Dr. McCoy, almost as an afterthought, that I had been having some back pain and had gone for a few treatments with my chiropractor. He told me maybe I should go for a bone scan since it had been several years since I had had one. I was thinking, "Well, it wouldn't hurt and at least it would help me rule out anything serious."

After I went for the bone scan, it would be almost a week before I went back to Dr. McCoy for the results. For a bone scan, they inject dye into your veins and you have to wait about two and a half hours until you actually have the scan. My husband and I left the hospital and got something to eat, did a little shopping, and then returned. Many thoughts went through my mind, but I tried not to think the worse.

The day I went back to Dr. McCoy for the results, I was a little apprehensive. My sister, Joyce, and my friend, Madeline went with me. I think they were more concerned than I was. After they called me in at the office, I told them they could stay in the waiting room. I really wasn't expecting bad news. As the nurse took me in to see the doctor, she went and brought them in, so I was getting a little nervous.

As he entered the room, I was sitting on the examining table. He came over and looked me straight in the eye and told me some places had showed up in my bones and the cancer medicine I was taking was no longer working and things were out of control again and we needed to get it back in control. My sister left the room. I knew why. He told me we would try some radiation again which should help the pain and then I would go back on chemo. Also, they would start me that day with a bone strengthening treatment called Zometa that would be given to me through my portacath. I am so glad I have kept my port in and not had it removed.

As of today, I have had 16 more radiation treatments which really helped the pain and I am still on chemo for maintenance. I had a lot of diarrhea when I took the radiation because it was directed in my pelvic area. I had to take medicine for that, too. I took ten radiation treatments, and then had to go back and take six more for the pain in my back which really helped. I thank God that He puts us with wonderful doctors who do not want to see us suffer or in pain and they will do all they can do to alleviate that. I have been so blessed with friends, family, doctors, and nurses who will always hold a special place in my heart.

I go through chemo about once a month and also have my Zometa with it. I get my blood checked the weeks in between. My white count goes down drastically, but I always bounce back and am able to take my treatments. I have some hair left, but I usually wear one of my pretty wigs when I go out. I'm used to them by now. I will be on this chemo as long as it is working and if it fails, we will try something else. I will always be on some kind of treatment, but I know I have to do this to survive. After all, what is the alternative? I know I am in God's hand and He will bring me "Through the Fire Again."

Afterthought

There is "life after cancer" and I cherish each day. I lost my precious Roy in October, 2009. Life is hard without my companion, but I feel God has left me here for a reason including writing this book. We weren't expecting to lose Roy when we did, but he got sick really fast and died in Roanoke Memorial Hospital peacefully with me and the boys around him. He was diagnosed with Pulmonary Fibrosis which is a lung disease that cuts off your oxygen and hardens your lungs. I have the assurance of knowing where he is, that I will see him again, and that we had those last two weeks with him to tell him all we needed to say, that he was loved.

www.ingramcontent.com/pod-product-compliance
Lightning Source LLC
Chambersburg PA
CBHW020352290526
45785CB00005B/2254